I0101551

Detox 3

Detoxify Your Body Gently the Natural Way

in 3 weeks

2nd edition 2017

Dr. Angela C. Fritz
Holistic Health Practitioner
&
Master Herbalist

>>><<<

Copyright © New Medical Frontiers, Inc. 2016

2nd edition 2017

ISBN: 978-0692638934

This is the second edition of this popular guide to detoxify your body gently the natural way. It has been updated with additional information on herbs and some more recipe ideas.

Contents

Disclaimer

The information given in this book is for informational purposes only and is not intended to replace the advice and treatment by a healthcare provider. All contents of this book are commentary or opinion and are protected under 'Free Speech' laws in all civilized countries. The information is provided for educational and entertainment purposes only and is not intended to diagnose, treat, cure, or prevent any condition or disease. Dr. Angela Fritz assumes no responsibility for the use or misuse of this material. No warranty of any kind, whether expressed or implied, is given in relation to this information or any of the external services referred to. This is a comprehensive limitation of liability that applies to all damages of any kind, including (without limitation) compensatory, direct, indirect or consequential damages.

Introduction: How to detoxify

Pollutants and contaminants from the environment are attacking our body, constantly. Our body absorbs a lot of toxins. Even if we try to watch our diet, we consume a lot of artificial preservatives and food additives.

Our body is made to fulfill the task of cleansing and purifying. Mostly, it is done in the liver, collecting waste and toxic elements, preparing to be removed from the body via bloodstream, colon and kidney, and perspiration. If this does not work properly, the liver gets overloaded and loses its ability to cleanse and purify. Our health is at stake, serious health problems may occur.

Therefore, we should detoxify and cleanse on a regular basis the natural way – natural and gentle. Aggressive pharmaceutical detox formulas often have side effects. It is much more efficient to rely on natural herbs in order to assist the body in obtaining its ability to eliminate waste and toxins.

Detoxifying does not mean changing your diet drastically. You do not have to only eat raw food or juice everything for some time. Don't choose a diet that lets you be hungry for weeks. Detoxifying is not abstinence of food, but rather being aware of what you eat, eating the right, healthy food, and using herbs to assist in the process. Beyond that, purifying in combination with herbs means fueling your body with new energy.

Proper detoxification has to include the whole body and all pathways, where toxins and waste are gathered and eliminated. For that rely on natural herbs to assist all parts of your body in obtaining its ability to detoxify.

In order to help your body in cleansing and purification process, you should focus on the following pathways to eliminate waste and in addition toxins.

Excreting:

Our colon should be cleansed on a regular basis.

The colon absorbs nutrients and discharges most of dietary fiber. The more you are able to excrete body waste, the greater is the chance to get rid of toxic substances as well.

Increasing Urination:

It's the job of our kidneys to cleanse and purify all liquids that are passing through. Whatever is not valuable to our body is elimitated. Encouraging dehydration leads to a bigger emission of toxic substances.

Perspiration:

Our skin is one of the body's pathways to eliminate waste and toxins by perspiration (sweating).

Detoxifying the natural way has three columns:

➢ **Nutrition** (particularly suitable for cleansing and purifying)

➢ **Herbs** (particularly ones acting as aid for cleansing and detoxifying) – including a "Detox Tea", that is blended to assist the body's ability to cleanse and purify , and

➢ **Physical Exercise**

Focus on these three columns for 3 weeks:

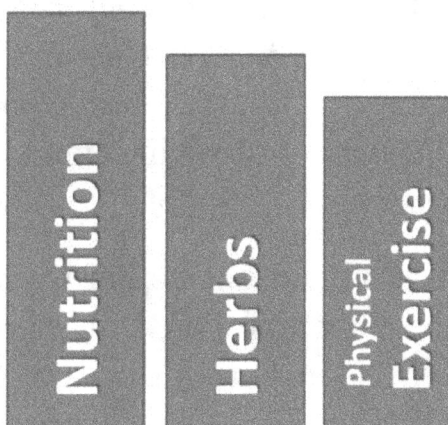

Nutrition   Herbs   Physical Exercise

Liver and kidneys play an important role in cleansing the body. These organs will be supported and strengthened by nutrients and herbs, we will introduce to, and a special "Detox Tea" blend.

This book is a handbook. It will give you instructions on how to detoxify and cleanse your body in three weeks in a gentle and natural way. The book should be your companion starting with analyzing and planning your food intake up to managing your personal detoxification process.

After you learn about the basics of detoxifying, and food and herbs that are vital in this process, structured work sheets will guide you first to get things straight concerning your food intake so far. In the next step, there will be guidance how to adjust your diet, creating your personal plan – involving food, herbs and physical exercise.

All in all it should not be hard work, but fun. That's the only way you will succeed. Try to stick to the plan longer than the suggested 3 weeks – this will be the foundation to a healthy, trim, and normal weight body.

Column #1: Nutrition

When it comes to food and diet, there are some simple general rules you should follow.

(1) As often as possible prepare your food yourself. Home cooking means you know what you eat – if you avoid processed food. Buy genuine natural ingredients that are not cooked, spiced, processed, or altered in any way.

(2) Get your nutrients from a variety of foods. The more different foods you include in your diet, the greater is the chance to get the most nutritional value.

(3) Use a lot of herbs to spice your food (and reduce salt). Herbs are good for your health, and: they pamper your taste buds. This way you will like to eat healthy even better.

(4) Choose whole grain over refined.

(5) Use fats – they help to enhance the taste of our food. But use fats sparsely and choose

non refined oils more often than butter. Substitute avocado for butter on your sandwich. Avoid 'trans fats'.

(6)   Food that has a lot of fiber helps to excrete waste. Some food and especially herbs are diuretic and help to drain your body. Bitters that you find in food and herbs (even, if you don't taste it) are important in order to stimulate all digestive organs. A lot of foods and herbs help to cleanse your liver and other organs. Most herbs help with digestion and to detoxify, cleanse, and purify your body.

In the next step we will introduce you to food groups first, later to especially valuable choices. The moment you are ready to create your personal plan, we want to make sure you include food you really like. That's the only way to stick to your plan and succeed.

Creating your personal plan means picking the foods you like best within specific food groups and adding as much of foods and herbs (spices) mentioned for detoxifying as possible. Don't hesitate to try something new as well! Don't just stick to the things you know. Be adventurous and creative.

Clustering food into groups may help you to choose a wide variety of healthy – and in our case detoxifying foods. Pick whatever you like from each group – as much and as often as recommended.

Important Food Groups
- Especially arranged for detoxifying

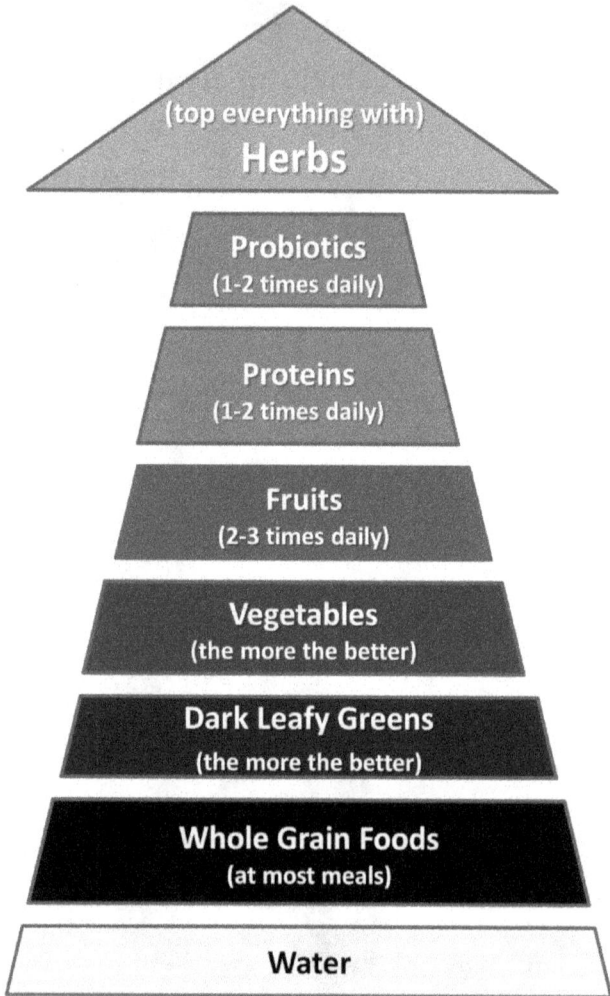

(top everything with)
Herbs

Probiotics
(1-2 times daily)

Proteins
(1-2 times daily)

Fruits
(2-3 times daily)

Vegetables
(the more the better)

Dark Leafy Greens
(the more the better)

Whole Grain Foods
(at most meals)

Water

✓ **Water** plays a big role when it comes to purifying your body. The body needs lots of liquids to wash out toxins and the best is water (spring water or filtered tab water).

✓ **Whole Grain Food** (whole wheat bread, whole wheat pasta, brown rice, old fashioned oats...). Whenever you eat grain: choose whole grain. Avoid refined grains, white flour and white rice. There are a lot of good nutrients in whole grain. In addition it contains the fiber you need for your digestion in order to excrete the waste.

✓ **Vegetables** are the big hit even before fruits. Prepared the right way (without cream or carbs, using just a little bit of olive oil and seasoned to your taste with herbs), you may eat as much as you like.

✓ **Dark Leafy Greens** (spinach, salad, kale ...) are part of the vegetable group. We have given this food a special extra place, because it is most important for detoxification. Dark Greens provide chlorophyll that helps to excrete environmental toxins. There is quite a variety to include green leaves in your diet: raw in salads, added to soup or veggies (raw and chopped), or sautéed with onions in olive oil, or blenderized added to juice.

✓ Seasoning is very important in order to please your taste buds. Only if you like to eat it, you will do so in abundance. Don't use a lot of salt, though. Try herbs and seeds to spice your food.

✓ **Fruits** come next. They are full of vitamins and especially antioxidants. Whenever you feel hungry: reach out for fruits. It's a good choice for a snack between meals. Especially berries: They are packed with antioxidants. Blueberries are best. Strawberries are a very good choice as well.

✓ **Proteins** are important as well, but to be consumed in moderation. Lean white meat (poultry), reduced fat dairy products, eggs, and fish should be part of your diet. (Eggs have regained their reputation in terms of health and as an energy provider). And don't forget about legumes: beans & lentils –

though vegetables – contain lots of proteins as well. That's why they are mentioned here.

✓ **Probiotics** are live bacteria your body needs in order to digest properly. They are found naturally in your body – your colon depends on these 'good bacteria' – and in certain foods. Consuming food that contains these 'good' bacteria will help most effectively in the process of cleansing and purifying. These bacteria help to move the food through your colon, and to digest the 'good' nutrients and eliminate the waste. Therefore probiotics are extremely important when it comes to detoxifying.

There are two common probiotic bacteria: **Lactobacillus** – found in dairy products and fermented foods (such as sauerkraut and fermented pickles) – and **Bifidobacterium** – found in some dairy products.

The easiest way to find these 'good' bacteria is **yogurt**. Yogurt has proteins as well, but is much more potent as a source of probiotics.

It promotes digestion and cares for a healthy colon. Be sure to read the label: It should say 'includes life active cultures' and at least mention Lactobacillus and Bifidobacterium – and no artificial additives. Choose 'plain' yogurt. It's better to add fruit and/or spices by yourself.

When looking for fermented food, choose 'barrel cured' sauerkraut to make sure it is not pasteurized. Pasteurization kills live active bacteria – also the good ones. Same goes for pickles. They have to be fermented. Salt and water - not vinegar - has to be used in the pickling process in order to grow the 'good' bacteria. In addition sauerkraut contains a lot of vitamins that help boost the immune system.

Even 'Hot Sauce', when made out of fermented chili peppers, is probiotic. Sour dough bread is a good source for probiotics as well. But again: Make sure it contains naturally grown 'sour dough'.

There are also **'prebiotic'** foods. Other than probiotics these foods do not contain live bacteria, but have the ability to feed the good bacteria that are already in your guts. Prebiotic foods are asparagus, artichokes, oats, and legumes as well as bananas, and honey. Even red wine is supposed to help good bacteria growth in your body. (Drink in moderation! 1 glass per day or less.)

✓ **Herbs** should top everything when it comes to detoxifying – used as spices, prepared as tea, or taken by mouth. There are a lot of herbs that help to drain and eliminate waste as well as to detoxify liver and other organs. We will introduce you to the most important ones in the next chapter.

Special Detox Foods
- help your body to detoxify

Foods that are listed in the next chapters should be on your list when it comes to cleansing your body. Use a lot of them. They will help to excrete toxins, encourage liver function, and increase bile production and urination.

As you may see there are a lot of veggies listed. Eat these as often as possible. All fruits are healthy as well and full of antioxidants, which fight free radicals and therefore help with cleansing and purifying – so eat a lot. Watch out especially for blueberries and strawberries.

Have a closer look at the great variety of herbs. Use them to spice your meals as often and as much as you can. Herbs help a lot with cleansing your liver and detoxify your body.

Specially Recommended Vegetables and Fruits

Artichoke, a member of the Milk Thistle family, is grown all over the world. The flower petals and fleshy flower bottoms are eaten as vegetable. Artichokes assist the liver to perform at its best, while clearing the body of toxins. They stimulate the production of bile fluid, which helps to extract nutrients, the body needs, properly. In addition artichokes contain a lot of fiber, magnesium, folic acid and potassium.

How to use best: If possible buy fresh artichokes. If not, canned in a jar (not can) is fine. Add to salads.

See also Artichoke leaf powder in "Special Detox Herbs".

Asparagus – is one of the most important foods when it comes to draining and with that detoxifying kidneys and bladder. Eat it steamed as a side to chicken breast. If you cook asparagus, do not discard the cooking water.

Use it in soup or your smoothie. It still contains valuable ingredients.

How to use best: Use fresh or frozen asparagus. Cook and eat as veggie or top your salad with it.

Avocado – has a lot of fiber and antioxidants and is therefore on our list of detoxifying foods. In addition avocados provide 'good fats' in abundance.

How to use best: Cut in half, remove the pit, cut in wedges and remove peel. Try to get everything that is directly underneath the peel: that part is packed with antioxidants. Cut into pieces and top your salad, or mash the pulp, adding finely chopped onions, lemon juice, a dash of salt and other herbs, if you like. Do not use prepared seasoning blends. Use as a spread on whole wheat bread. Try to substitute butter or mayonnaise by mashed avocado on your sandwich.

Beets – are a very important element in any detox diet. They support the detoxifying and cleansing process. Beets contain a lot of vitamins (A, B1, B2, B6, C), folic acid, lots of minerals and fiber. They are considered a blood cleanser.

How to use best: Cook beets as a whole. They are easily to peel after cooking and do not 'bleed out' this way. Let cool, peel, and cut into bite size pieces. Marinade with a mix of lemon, salt, and other herbs you like. You may use mustard as well. But read the label: It should only mention mustard seeds, vinegar, and maybe turmeric. No other additives or preservatives. Eat beets cold as a salad of its own or put it in your salad, or eat warm as a side dish.

Bitter Melon – is native to Asia, but grows well in tropical climates of South America, today. The fruit is harvested before ripening and looks a little bit like a cucumber. It is a good source of vitamin C and vitamin A, phosphorus, and iron. After ripening it changes color and becomes bitterer. Containing insulin-like peptides, Bitter Melon has a long tradition to be used to regulate blood glucose levels. Modern research, clinical trials, confirm Bitter Melons efficacy on diabetes. Furthermore,

Bitter Melon has shown to lower total cholesterol, triglycerides, and LDL and increase levels of HDL, and to reduce body fat.

The reason Bitter Melon is mentioned here is the observation that it protects and enhances liver function. It has an antioxidant capacity to scavenge free radicals. Therefore Bitter Melon will help you cleanse your liver.

How to use best: You may add Bitter Melon to your diet, if you like the bitter taste. In Asian cooking it is mostly stir-fried in a wok. If not: add ½ to 1 Tsp. (not more – don't overdose) Bitter Melon powder to a drink or to your oatmeal. The powder of the fruit does not taste bitter, usually. But be careful and make sure to buy genuine fruit powder. Supplement capsules often contain seed and leaf in addition to fruit. Seed and leaf are not as safe as fruit and may have side effects. Be careful, if you are on any medication for diabetes. The efficacy could be enhanced.

Blueberries – are great antioxidants and supposed to help not only live healthier, but longer. A growing number of studies suggest that blueberries help organs to function properly and boost fat and glucose burning.

How to use best: Eat blueberries raw, not cooked in a pie or muffin. If you can't get fresh blueberries, frozen are fine – they thaw on the kitchen counter in no time. Eat just plain or add to yogurt or oats.

Broccoli – a super food everyone has heard about. But why is it on the list of foods for detoxifying? Constituents in broccoli work together with liver enzymes, especially, in order to transform toxins into something the body is easier able to excrete.

How to use best: Add raw broccoli florets to your salad or eat as a snack. For a quick side dish cook frozen broccoli florets in a steam bag in your microwave. Don't like broccoli? Season it! Or try it with a quick cheese sauce, stirring hot water into softened fat reduced cream cheese.

Cabbage – helps to cleanse the liver, stimulates digestion and is therefore an essential aide when it comes to detoxifying.

25

Besides that, cabbage is known to lower cholesterol. For variety look out to the whole 'cabbage family' including Brussels sprouts and bok choy.

How to use best: Cabbage can be used any way you like, cooked as a side, shredder raw for salads. Use any herb or spice for seasoning. Seeds like cumin and caraway go well with it. Try it also seasoned with turmeric, a dash of cayenne pepper, and soya sauce.

Onions – are an all present bulb in every kitchen, providing taste to food that should not contain too much salt. Onions are packed with amino acids containing sulfur, which efficiently detoxifies the liver. Health benefits of raw onions are higher. Make sure to include some in your diet, daily. Try red onions. They are not as pungent as yellow ones.

Strawberries – have significant health benefits and have been studied well because of their anti-cancer, anti-microbial, and anti-oxidant activities as well as their ability to regulate blood sugar.

How to use best: Same as blueberries (and all other berries) eat strawberries raw. If fresh strawberries are not in season, look into the freezer. Do not use sugar to sweeten, try stevia powdered leaves instead, if desired.

Fluids

Water – should be the basis of every detox diet. It is very important for all organs to flush out toxins. While exercising and taking saunas to help release the toxins it is very important to stay hydrated. Please be careful: If your body is not used to drinking a lot of water, be sure to only increase your intake slowly, day by day. This way your kidneys can get used to extended flushing. And don't forget to restore your body with minerals that are flushed out. Spring water contains minerals. And a lot of herbs and especially seeds contain minerals, too. Make sure to include these in your daily diet.

Green Tea – is a perfect addition for every detox diet. It has a high antioxidant value. Antioxidants help seek out and kill free radicals before they can do any damage.

Green Tea is the same plant as black tea. The leaves are processed in a different way that preserves the integrity of the nutrients. Especially polyphenols, that are believed to be responsible for the antioxidant activity of Green Tea, stay intact.

Research suggests that regular Green Tea drinkers may have a lower risk of developing heart disease and certain types of cancer. Latest studies suggest the effect of Green Tea consumption on weight-loss maintenance.

Because of its high antioxidant value, we have made Green Tea the basic ingredient of our "Detox Tea".

Lemon – yes, we have listed it under "fluids": You should drink it with water. Lemon contains vitamin C, which helps the body to excrete toxins and burn fat. Lemon juice with water - hot or cold – washes out toxins. Drink one glass or cup in the morning before breakfast. That will help to stimulate digestion and especially liver function. It is a proven remedy to alkalize the body.

Lemon is actually a super fruit in disguise. Add the juice to water and create a wonder drink that nourishes and hydrates your body, boosts your energy, and may even help you losing weight. Drink lemon water before breakfast and it will help you detoxify and regulate your metabolism. There are - at least - 11 reasons to make it a habit to drink lemon water.

11 good reasons to make drinking lemon water a habit

Nutrients: Lemon has a lot of nutritional value. It is low in calories and a good source for vitamin C and folate, as well as potassium, calcium, and magnesium.

PH-value: Lemon water creates an alkaline effect in your body and raises your PH-value. Studies show that the higher your PH-value, the better your body is able to fight illnesses.

Detox: Lemon water in the morning stimulates your whole metabolism. It encourages your liver to set toxins free, cleanses your liver, and stimulates bile production. In addition it cleanses blood and arteries. This way it is one of the best things to do for detoxifying your body.

Digestion and bowl movement: Lemon water in the morning encourages bowl movement.

Weight loss: Lemon water may help you losing weight, helping burn more fat and calories. Drink lemon water before every meal.

Skin: Lemon is a strong antioxidant that fights free radicals. In addition ascorbic acid helps your skin to be more elastic and have a youthful and healthy glow.

Depression and anxiety: Due to its high level of potassium, lemon water may even help with anxiety and depression. Both are often causes by potassium deficit.

Infections: Lemon has an anti-inflammatory effect and helps to fight infections.

Gout: Lemon water dilutes uric acid and washes out toxins, this way helping with gout.

Heart Burn: Due to its alkaline effect, lemon water may help with acid reflux.

How to use best: Lemon water in the morning is best for your body, if it is warm - not hot and not cold. Heat will destroy valuable vitamins.

For the purpose of drinking lemon water before breakfast, heat water to a point that it feels warm to your fingertips. Add juice of 1/2 lemon to one cup of water. Sweeten with honey or stevia, if you like and drink slowly.

During the day drink lemon water as homemade 'lemonade' - cold and with ice, if you like.

Don't wait to make drinking lemon water a habit!

Column # 2: Herbs

'Herb' is called every part of a plant (root, bark, leave, stalk, flower, seed ..., or the whole plant). The original Latin word 'herba' stands for 'leave', 'plant, 'meadow' as well as (medicinal) herb and remedy. Most of the herbs, we will introduce you to, you may use as spices in your food, some are better consumed as tea, and some you should just take by mouth because of its medicinal value.

Medicinal herbs – like Milk Thistle, Bitter Melon fruit powder (mentioned above), and Artichoke leaf powder – are taken because of the medicinal efficacy. You have to be careful, if you are taking any pharmaceutical drugs having the same efficacy. But don't be hesitant either. These herbs may be the better alternative. Just follow dosage recommendations.

Make sure to buy whole herbs, not extracts. The whole herb usually has constituents that help your body to digest properly. Extracts may have side effects that whole herbs do not have. Do not go for capsules. You never know what's exactly in it. And make sure to buy herbs that are fresh and do not have a long shelf life.

Relying on herbs is the basis of a natural, smooth and healthy detoxifying process. Supplements that promote harsh bowl-evacuation and/or strong diuretics deprive the body of vital nutrients and minerals. In order to eliminate waste and toxic residues, reach for herbs that are gentle. In the following we will introduce you to most effective ones (in alphabetic order).

Special Detox Herbs

- help your body to detoxify

Annatto - is the seed of the Achiote tree that grows in tropical and subtropical regions all over the world. It is commonly used in Latin American and Caribbean cuisines. It has a slightly nutty, sweet and peppery (not hot) flavor.

Research suggests annatto protects liver, lowers blood pressure & cholesterol. Traditionally it is used to tone, balance, and strengthen the liver, to lower high cholesterol, as a strong diuretic, for high blood pressure, and for heartburn.

How to use best: Annatto's slight nutty taste blends well in sweet dishes as well as salty ones. To make use of the flavonoides provided by the very bright red color, always add a little bit of fat. Give it a try! Add it to your oats in the morning or your veggies during the day.

Artichoke *leaf powder*

We covered artichokes under "special detox foods" already: The flower petals and fleshy flower bottoms are eaten as vegetable. The plant chemical "cynarin", however, is found in high concentration in the green parts of the plant, mainly the leaves. Cynarin is considered one of artichoke's main biologically active chemicals. Research confirms that cynarin lowers high cholesterol (LDL), increases bile production, and detoxifies and protects the liver. Most recent studies note that artichoke leafs may even reverse liver damage done by harmful chemicals.

How to use best: Artichoke leaf powder tastes bitter. Therefore the best ways to take it is, stirring it into some pleasant tasting food like orange juice or apple sauce – and take it as a bitter medicine. Recommended dosage is ½ Tsp up to 2 times daily. Using the whole herb and not an extract will include other active chemicals of the plant that may assist the efficacy.

Celery seeds - have marked liver protective activity. Used as a tea or cooked in soup these seeds support the cleansing process and help to disinfect the bladder. Celery seeds are therefore used for treating rheumatic conditions and gout. Because of its great value for cleansing and purifying, we have included celery seeds in our "Detox Tea".

How to use best: Add celery seeds to every meal you want to. For best nutritional value cook celery seeds or drink as a tea: ¼ tsp. per cup of water, bring to a boil and let simmer for at least 5 minutes.

Cumin & Caraway – are two different plants. Cumin originates in North Africa and caraway in Europe. But both seeds have similar efficacies. Both are traditionally used for illnesses of the digestive system, reducing gases and abdominal distension. Research suggests that both stimulate the entire digestive process. Therefore it is good to include those seeds in your diet, especially when detoxifying your body. In addition both seeds are a good source of protein, vitamin C, magnesium, phosphorus, potassium, zinc, copper and manganese, and a very good source of dietary fiber, calcium and iron.

How to use best: These seeds are hard, so it is best to use them in cooked food. If you do not like to bite on it: use (freshly) ground or put the seeds in a tea strainer or muslin bag and take it out after cooking. For freshness grind seeds by yourself, using a coffee grinder or just your blender. This way you may use more, even in salad dressing.

Dandelion – is thought of as a weed, but has remarkable health benefits. Traditionally it is used as a diuretic and detoxifying remedy.

Research confirmed in 1974 that dandelion leaves are a powerful diuretic. Since the leaves contain high levels of potassium it counteracts the side effect of loosing potassium while draining. (Conventional diuretics deprive the body of minerals, especially potassium.) Dandelion is a good source of folate, magnesium, phosphorus, and copper, and a very good source of dietary fiber, vitamin A, vitamin C, vitamin E (alpha tocopherol), vitamin K, thiamin, riboflavin, vitamin B6, calcium, iron, potassium and manganese. This way dandelion provides a lot of nutrients the body is losing when drained.

Because dandelion is vital for detoxifying, we have included it in our "Detox Tea".

How to use best: Add fresh, young dandelion leaves to your salad (make sure the meadow has not been sprayed with chemicals!). If you do not live in an area, where dandelion grows, or in winter time: substitute fresh for dried leaves. The effect is the same. Sprinkle over your salad.

Fennel seeds – are traditionally used for illnesses of the digestive system. Research suggests Fennel seeds to relieve bloating, and settle stomach pain. Fennel seeds are diuretic and anti-inflammatory – and therefore a good choice to be included in a detoxifying diet.

Like almost all seeds, fennel seeds are a good source of minerals – like phosphorus, potassium, copper, calcium, iron, magnesium and manganese, as well as a very good source of dietary fiber.

How to use best: You may add fennel to all cooked food or use it ground in salad dressings or in your oatmeal. (Use coffee grinder or blender for grinding.) A good choice to use fennel is also to drink it as a tea – combined with other herbs and seeds for detoxifying.

Flax seeds – is traditionally used as a potent laxative, especially valuable in chronic constipation. Research has found high level of omega-3 fatty acid (similar to fish oil) and indicates that (ground or crushed) flax seed has cancer fighting activity.

How to use best: There are two ways. As a laxative, you take a spoon full of kernels (swallow whole) and drink at least 5 times their volume of water. If you hit for the omega 3 value, sprinkle a spoon full over your cereal and try to chew every little seed. Make sure to drink a lot, when eating flax seeds.

Garlic – has a long tradition as remedy and medicinal herb, to protect against infections, as well as to stimulate circulation and to thin blood.

Research shows that garlic also helps to lower high blood fat levels, high blood pressure, and high blood sugar levels, and that it has an antibiotic activity. It may even prevent circulatory problems and stroke.

How to use best: Add garlic to every food you like, chopped or crushed. Raw is best, but cooked is better than not.

Note: The medically active constituent in garlic, Allicin, is not ready in a whole clove and not heat resistant. Allicin, is created while garlic is chopped, crushed, or pressed. Make sure to wait 10 minutes before heating.

Extra hint: Chew a few kernels of coriander seeds. These are traditionally used to sweeten breath especially after eating garlic.

Ginger – is known as a healing root since ancient Chinese times. It stimulates circulation and regulates blood pressure. In addition ginger assists the liver in eliminating "free radicals".

Detox 3 - Detoxify Your Body the Natural Way

How to use best: Use fresh or ground dried ginger in any food you like. Put it in tea or simply brew it with hot water as a beverage of its own.

Lemon Grass – is used traditionally as a natural way to cleanse several organs – such as liver, kidneys, bladder, and the entire digestive tract. Better circulation and better digestion are benefits of this herb as well. Because of its virtue for all vital organs, we have included this herb in our "Detox Tea".

How to use best: Especially dried lemon grass is hard. If used for cooking, it is a good idea to put it in your blender before adding to food. This will chop the hard pieces and will unfold the exquisite aroma. Use in your salads and with chicken or all kind of veggies.

Milk Thistle – is not a spice, but a very important herb to help to detoxify your liver.

Medicinal benefits of milk thistle have been valued for more than 2,000 years. It has been used since the Middle Ages to improve liver function.

Scientific research confirms milk thistle to actually help with liver disease treatment and prevention. It is used primarily to help with dyspeptic complaints and liver conditions, including toxin-induced liver damage and hepatic cirrhosis, and as a supportive therapy for chronic inflammatory liver conditions.

How to use best: Cook one tsp. of whole seeds in water. Eat the seeds and drink the water. Or use ground seeds (no extracts). Either pour a cup of boiling water over one teaspoon of ground seeds, steep for 10-20 minutes. Or take milk thistle seeds by mouth in a dose of 1 tsp of fresh ground seeds daily – stir into a little amount of food (apple sauce, yogurt, mashed potatoes) or juice (orange juice).

Parsley – is highly nutritious and may be considered a natural vitamin and mineral supplement by itself. The seeds have stronger diuretic actions and are used like celery seeds in the treatment of gout, rheumatism, and arthritis. Seeds of both plants (parsley and celery) – prepared as tea or cooked in soup –

encourage the flushing out of waste products and toxins.

One cup parsley provides 101% daily value of vitamin A, 133% daily value of vitamin C, 1230% daily value of vitamin K, and a very good source of Dietary Fiber, Folate, Calcium, Iron, Magnesium, Potassium, Copper and Manganese, and is a good source of Protein, Vitamin E (Alpha Tocopherol), Thiamin, Riboflavin, Niacin, Vitamin B6, Pantothenic Acid, Phosphorus and Zinc.

Leaves, seeds and root are used in herbal medicine – leaves mostly for the nutritional value, seeds and root as a diuretic to flush out waste and to promote menstruation. Leaves contain volatile oils that relieve cramps and flatulence as well as flavonoids that are anti-oxidant and anti-inflammatory.

How to use best: Chop fresh parsley and add to every meal, if possible: salads, veggies, potatoes, you name it. Always add at the very last minute. Do not cook fresh parsley. Vital vitamins will be destroyed.

Extra hint: Grow your own fresh parsley.

Parsley grows in every garden and climate. If you live in areas with hot summers, choose to grow parsley in fall. Grow your own parsley in a pot. This way you will be able to change its location to more or less sun. Like all herbs parsley grows stronger outside, exposed to sun and fresh air. Grow from seeds or buy plants at a farmers market, not in a super market. Cut leaves as frequently as you desire, they will grow back. Parsley even needs 'a haircut' once in a while to grow strong. If the plant brings out flowers, let them bloom and convert into seeds. Use the seeds in soups or brew a tea – to flush out toxins.

Turmeric – is a powerful anti-inflammatory herb and has a long tradition as a remedy to help improve liver function. The yellow ingredient curcuma increases bile production, lowers cholesterol and has a protective action on stomach and liver. There is encouraging research that turmeric may be a valuable preventive remedy for the risk of developing cancer.

More about this yellow root:
Turmeric is a perennial plant of the ginger family, which is native to southwest India. The roots are dried and ground into a yellow powder. It's a basic ingredient in Indian cooking and common in Asian cuisine as well. It has a slightly bitter, earthy taste that does not disturb any other flavor.

Besides in cooking, Turmeric has been used as a remedy - traditionally in Ayurvedic and Chinese medicine to treat inflammatory conditions, skin diseases, wounds, digestive ailments and liver conditions.

Some decades ago western researcher noticed that India has some of the lowest rates of colon, prostate and lung cancer in the world. This advantage was traced largely to the diet that includes consistent intake of turmeric.

Today we know that naturally occurring phytochemicals, referred to as curcuminoids, provide not only the yellow color, but many health benefits. Turmeric has anti-oxidant, anti-septic and anti-inflammatory properties.

Here are some findings of latest research.

Turmeric's anti-oxidant and anti-inflammatory properties may play a key role in preventing and treating a lot of chronic diseases.

Curcuma increases bile production, helping improve liver function and has a protective action on stomach and liver.

There is encouraging research that turmeric may be a valuable preventive remedy for the risk of developing cancer.

Turmeric is used in clinical studies as a natural anti-inflammatory treatment.

Early studies suggest that turmeric may lower cholesterol and may help prevent the build-up of plaque in the arteries.

How to use best: Use as often as possible. Turmeric hardly tastes of anything (only if you use too much, it may taste bitter). Therefore you may use it in any food you do not mind that it turns yellow – in rice as well as in your morning cereal. See also recipe ideas.

Detox Tea

Fluids – as mentioned above – are vital to flush out toxins. Add herbs that help purifying your body and cleansing your liver to hot water. This will provide a drink – "Detox Tea" – that is essential part of a detoxifying diet. It will support you efforts to detoxify your body.

To prepare herbs as herbal teas always has a specific benefit. Constituents that have special medicinal values are better released, if brewed with hot water. If you use dried herbs, use boiling water and let steep for a few minutes. If you use seeds, it is best to bring to a boil and let simmer for a few minutes.

Herbs often used for detoxifying teas are ginger, celery seeds, and lemon grass.

The Herbery (www.yourherbery.com) has created a special blend that assists in the cleansing process. Our "Detox Tea" contains Green Tea, celery seeds, dandelion, ginger, lemon citric acid, lemon grass, milk thistle, and Pau d' Arco.

As mentioned before, **Green Tea** has a high antioxidant value, **Celery** seeds are diuretic and help cleansing the body, **Dandelion** is diuretic and detoxifying, and adds vital minerals, **Ginger** helps with liver function, **Lemon** citric acid flushes out toxins, **Lemon Grass** helps to cleanse liver, kidneys and bladder.

Since scientific research confirms that **Milk Thistle** actually helps, when the liver is overwhelmed by toxins, we have added this herb as well. As mentioned before, milk thistle has been used since ancient times to improve liver function.

We have added **Pau d'Arco** as well. Pau d' Arco is a big tree native to the Amazon rainforest. The inner bark is used for medicinal purposes. Research suggests that Pau d'Arco fights free radicals and cleanses the blood.

All these herbs complement each other in the process of purifying and cleansing. The combination of herbs in our "Detox Tea" also improves digestion and helps to remove waste that is hindering absorption of good nutrients from your diet.

During the period of three weeks this tea should be on your menu at least 3 times a day.

For more information go to
http://www.yourherbery.com/store/p131/Detox_Tea.html

Column # 3: Physical Exercise

Perspiration is one of the body's pathways to eliminate waste and toxins.

The skin is our biggest organ. You absorb toxic substances through your skin the same way you may absorb well doing ingredients – applied as ointment or in a nice hot bath, when you add herbs to your bath water. The other way around, you are able to eliminate toxic substances by perspiration.

The benefit of cleansing and purifying the body by perspiration has been known since ancient times. There were hot steaming sweat baths – similar to "saunas" we know in our days.

An even better way to get rid of toxic substances through your skin is 'sweating' while physical exercising. The advantage of physical exercise is that your whole circulation is stimulated. This way more toxic substances – especially from organs like your liver – may be transported to places where they can be excreted – your skin, your kidneys and bladder, and your colon.

Exercise and sport help to boost circulation and bring all organs to life. This way it helps to get rid of body wastes by perspiring toxins through our skin. The body works much more efficient with physical exercise. Therefore it is vital to try to include 30 minutes of sweat inducing exercise (at least almost) daily in your personal plan.

If you are not used to it, start slowly, but be persistent. Don't listen to your body, telling you to quit. Start with brisk walking, proceeding to running. You have to find exercise that makes you perspire.

Your Personalized Plan

Every human being is different and has a different metabolism. Therefore it is very important to have a **personalized** plan for detoxifying your body.

The following graphic gives you an idea how it works.

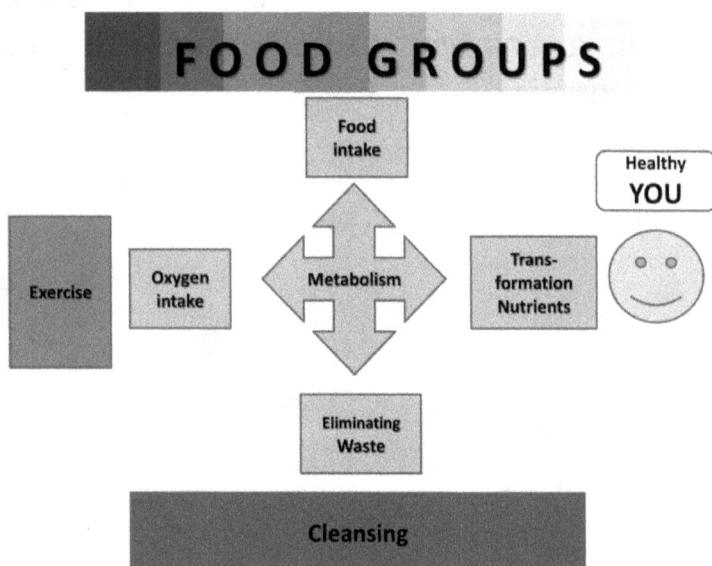

FOOD GROUPS

Food intake

Healthy
YOU

Exercise

Oxygen intake

Metabolism

Trans-formation Nutrients

Eliminating Waste

Cleansing

Your metabolism is determined by food intake (eating nutrients), oxygen intake (breathing), transforming good nutrients into energy, and eliminating waste. Pay attention to your food (by using food groups), exercise in order to get a lot of oxygen; cleanse your body in order to get rid of waste. All this will help to transform good nutrients properly and will finally lead to a healthy "You".

Foods and herbs that help with detoxifying will boost your metabolism. Boosting your metabolism means burning more fat and getting more nutrients out of your food.

Pick your food from the food groups that were listed in chapter "*Important Food Groups*", considering what you like. Make sure your body gets enough oxygen (physical exercise). The right intake of food and oxygen will lead to transform food into valuable nutrients on one hand and get rid of the waste the body does not need on the other hand.

Three Steps to Your Personalized Plan

Step 1: *Take a Survey*

Keep a diary for one week: What do you eat and when? How much and what do you drink? How much do you exercise? Be as precise and honest as possible.

Write down everything the moment after you have eaten, or drunken it. Do not try to remember in the evening or (worse) after a few days. List every ingredient you know of. Read the labels. Mark it, if you have had a home cooked meal or eaten out.

Step 2: _Analyze your diet and daily routine._

✓ Mark everything **red** that is processed, contains a lot of fat, salt, refined sugar, refined flour, or white rice. Mark everything **green** that is home cooked and fits into the food groups.

✓ Make a list of food you like to eat.

✓ Check these foods:

Food	Like a lot	Like a little	Don't like
Artichokes			
Asparagus			
Avocado			
Beets			
Bitter Melon			
Broccoli			
Cabbage			
Onions			
Blueberries			
Strawberries			

✓ Check these herbs:

Herbs	Like a lot	Like a little	Don't like
Annatto			
Caraway			
Celery seeds			
Cumin			
Dandelion			
Fennel seeds			
Flax seeds			
Garlic			
Ginger			
Lemon Grass			
Parsley			
Turmeric			

✓ Make a list of exercise options you like to do / would like to do that could fit into your daily routine.

Step 3: _Create your healthy personal food plan for the next 3 weeks – using tools that follow._

Food Groups along the Day

Start your day

Before breakfast drink a glass of lemon water: Juice of ½ a lemon in 8 oz. of water – hot or cold. This detoxifies, assists your liver and helps with bowl movement. If you want to sweeten the drink, use stevia (genuine leaves are best) or honey, no sugar.

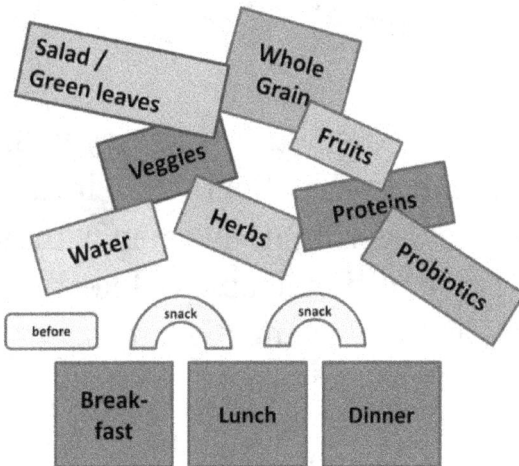

Breakfast

Try to eat a lot of healthy foods and herbs for breakfast. Your body needs energy in the morning.

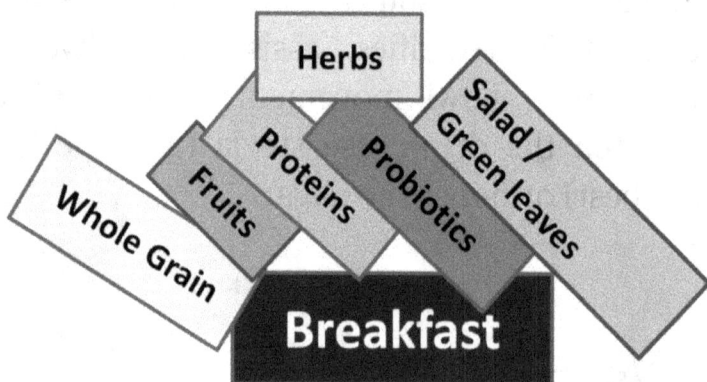

You like it sweet? Then start your day with oats and (probiotics) yogurt. Soak oats in a small amount of water overnight. Sweeten with honey or stevia. Try additional spices like turmeric and annatto, and add as much fruit as you like.

You do not like sweets? Try to spice your oats with herbs and a dash of salt.

Like it more savory? How about whole wheat toast with fat reduced cream cheese, spinach and some onions? Or substitute cream cheese for avocado and add one slice of fat reduced (chicken) bologna.

For drink: Replace your usual coffee with "Detox Tea". In addition you may try an "Herbal Energy Drink", containing herbs that have natural caffeine, increase stamina and lift up your spirits. Green Tea is a good choice as well.

("Herbal Energy Drink" is available at http://www.yourherbery.com/store/p53/Herbal_Energy_Drink.html)

Lunch

Try to have a relaxed lunch so you can enjoy your meal. Always plan a salad for lunch time. You are not eating at home? Make a salad your main meal for lunch time.

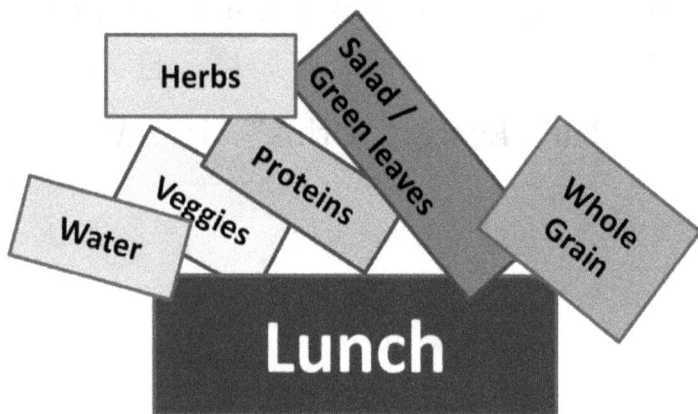

Pack all ingredients including dressing ready to eat, separately. Try to include as many detoxifying foods as possible (precooked beets, broccoli, avocado, and some shredded cabbage – whatever you like). And do not forget to include detoxifying herbs & spices in your dressing. Take along a bowl to mix everything.

You eat lunch at home? Settle for salad **and** veggies. Veggies do not have to be fresh. Frozen is good as well. Don't have a lot of time? Choose "steam bags" from the freezer that cook in microwave in minutes.

How about a spinach salad, followed by brown rice with steamed salmon and peas? Don't forget about turmeric and parsley!

To drink: Water is fine. Better is "Detox Tea" or a tea made with ginger and/or celery seeds. After lunch: Try a metabolic booster (Green Tea with lemon grass and ginger).

("Metabolic Booster" is available at

http://www.yourherbery.com/store/p68/Metabolic_Booster.html)

Dinner

Dinner should be light, not a big meal and if possible before 6 pm. Again you should eat salad and veggies. If you had a warm cooked meal at lunch, choose something cold – but do not forget the veggies.

Add raw broccoli florets, cooked asparagus, artichokes, and cooked beets to a big salad. Include more herbs (dandelion, garlic, ginger, annatto, and turmeric). Prepare vinaigrette made with olive oil, red wine vinegar and herbs. If you like, you may add mustard – but read the label: Only ingredients should be mustard seeds and vinegar; turmeric may be added.

Herbs

Salad /
Green Leaves

Whole Grain

Fruits

Veggies

Water

Proteins

Dinner

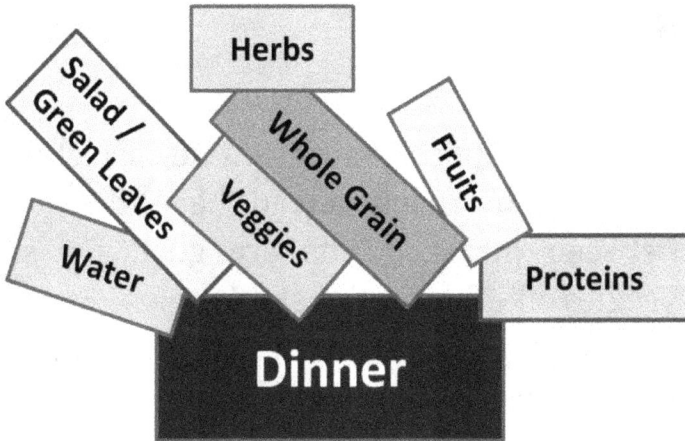

To drink: If you are sensitive to caffeine and have difficulty sleeping, skip the last cup "Detox Tea" and settle for water or a tea made with celery seeds. If not, you may add another cup of "Detox Tea" in the evening.

Trouble sleeping? Try a gentle herbal tea like "Sweeter Dreams" (Sweeter Dreams is available at http://www.yourherbery.com/store/p100/Sweeter_Dreams_.html)

Snacks

It is very important that you never feel hungry. Plan healthy snacks ahead, have them at hand between meals. Fruits are good for snacks, veggies like broccoli, celery stalks, carrots are even better. Berries are great. Probiotics are a good choice as well. Some low fat cheese is fine.

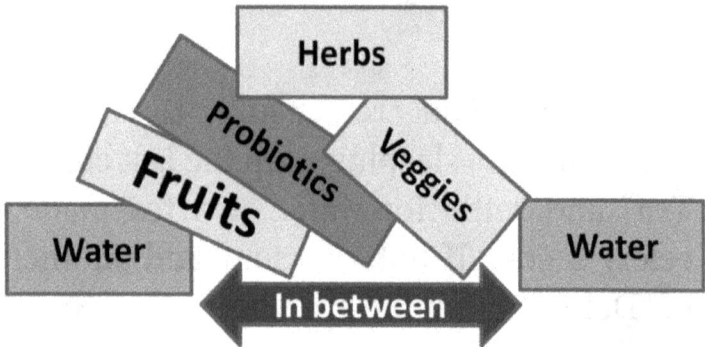

And make sure to drink a lot of water in between, during the day.

Drinks

Especially during times of a detox diet, you should drink a lot. That helps your body to flush out toxic substances. But be careful: If your body is not used to drink a lot, start with the amount you usually drink, adding an additional 8 oz. glass per day – until you reach the amount of about 8 glasses, teas, water, everything you drink included.

Pure water is always best. In times of a detox diet, you should include "Detox Tea", lemon water, Green Tea and teas made with ginger and celery seeds. You may drink everything cold or hot – just as you like it.

We recommend drinking "Detox Tea" at least 3 times a day.

Avoid hard liquor alcohol during this 3 weeks period of detoxifying your body. You may include some wine, if your body is content with some alcohol.

One glass of wine per day, red preferred, is considered healthy. The process of pressing and maturing red wine provides nutrients that act as 'prebotics', nourishing the 'good' bacteria in your guts. In addition 'resveratrol', found in red wine, coming from the red skins of the grapes, is supposed to have antioxidants and is helpful with several metabolic diseases.

Do not drink more than this single glass of red wine. Drinking more means adding calories, unnecessarily. And: drinking more in the evening may disrupt your sleep quality.

Create Your Personalized Plan

a) Take your list of favorite foods. Mark everything that does not fit into the food groups. Try to find other foods to substitute these.

b) Plan ahead the first week: What will you eat when? Breakfast / lunch / dinner and 2 snacks in between. You should not eat more than you did before. Only eat when you are hungry. Try to have small portions – more in the morning, less in the evening – if possible no later than 6 pm. *Write down everything in order to structure your day.*

c) Be sure to focus on picking and including special detoxifying foods and herbs as described.

d) Add at least 3 cups of "Detox Tea" per day. Since Green Tea contains a small amount of caffeine, do not drink it less than 2 hours before bedtime.

If you live in a family with kids and other adults, who have different needs in terms of food and cooking, you will have to adjust to the "family plan". All foods and herbs recommended are healthy for every human being. So, include detox food and herbs in the family food plan, adding more to your own meals and less carbs for yourself.

e) Add physical exercise to your plan. Try to include 30 min of **sweat-inducing exercise** at least 3 times a week, better every day.

Find the best way to include exercise in your daily schedule. For some it may be the time in the morning, just before breakfast. Others will like to unwind while running after a full day. If kids and family are demanding, try to split up 30 min to 3 times 10 min and spread out your workout time over the day.

Some more hints

➤ Plan at least one week ahead. This way you can make sure everything you want to eat is stocked up in your fridge or pantry.

➤ Try to include a big variety of food using as many detox foods as possible.

➤ Try to follow your taste buds: Only if you like what you eat, you can make sure you will stick to the diet.

➤ Detoxifying food will lead to increased urination. Make sure you plan your day ahead, including restroom stops.

➤ Problem with bowel movement? Eat more fiber and probiotics. Drink more water. Try natural things like swallowing 1 spoon of flax seeds (whole) with at least 5 times the amount of water.

➤ Use a lot of herbs to spice your meals – especially those, which help with detoxifying. Use salt sparsely. Do not use seasoning blends with salt. It's better to add salt by yourself. That way you will know how much salt is added.

➤ Don't like veggies? Season with herbs as much as you like. You may even sweeten veggies. But do not use sugar. Try genuine stevia instead.

➤ To sweeten always try to use genuine stevia (not extract) – dried crushed or powdered leaves – or buy your own stevia plant and use the leaves. Stevia leaves are very sweet, do not have any calories and provide extra minerals.

➤ Not much time to cook? Rely on your freezer and microwave: Use frozen veggies in a microwaveable steam bag. In 4 – 5 minutes you will have cooked veggies, you just have to season.

➤ Fill your freezer with veggies and quick to cook meats (like chicken breast).

➢ Cook meat ahead and freeze in appropriate portions. Use not only as center part of your meal, but with veggies in casseroles, stews, and in sandwiches.

➢ Use instant brown rice. It's ready in 10 minutes. Whole wheat couscous is a good choice as well. It's precooked (whole) wheat, ready in a few minutes.

➢ Stock your pantry with herbs and especially seeds. Seeds have a lot of minerals your body needs especially in times of elimination of toxins. Make sure to buy fresh (they should not have been sitting on a shelf for a long time)!

Planning Schedule

To plan your three weeks of detoxification, you have to plan your food intake as well as your exercise. Try to structure your *new* healthy daily routine.

Follow these steps:

1. Start with planning a typical day as an example – having in mind your personal (timely) needs during a 'normal' day, considering whether you have the chance to cook and eat at home, how much time you will have to prepare food and for exercise.

2. Make a rough plan for a 'normal' week.

3. Step back and look at your plans: Where is potential to improve – according to the suggestions in this book.

4. Plan your first week – day by day.

5. Decide what to prepare ahead and when. Include the evening to prepare for next day.

Invite a friend to join you during your effort to detoxify. Check, recheck, and talk about your plans. Encourage one another. It's much more easy than doing it all by yourself.

Some Quick Recipe Ideas

Oats for breakfast

Soak ½ cup of oats in water (just barely covered) overnight. Add 5 tablespoons yogurt, ¼ tsp. annatto, turmeric, honey or stevia to taste, and add cut up fruits like banana, apple, berries – or whatever is in season and you like to eat.

Quick and healthy sandwiches

(1) Take 2 slices of whole wheat or sour dough bread. Spread both with fat reduced cream cheese (Neufchatel), add thinly sliced onions and heap with spinach. Combine to a face closed sandwich.

(2) Take one slice of whole wheat or sour dough bread, mash 1/8 or ¼ avocado – depending on size – to spread on, add thinly sliced onion, 1 slice fat reduced (chicken) bologna and top with lots of spinach.

Quick Broccoli & Cheese

(1) Steam one bag of frozen broccoli florets in microwave (in microwaveable steam bag) 4 to 5 min.

(2) In a microwave safe bowl add 4 oz fat reduced cream cheese (Neufchatel) with 1 cup of water. Microwave for 30 seconds, whisk together until smooth (add another 30 seconds, if necessary).

(3) Grate 2 oz of cheese (which ever you prefer) and whisk into cream cheese sauce until dissolved.

(4) Combine broccoli and cheese sauce.

Broccoli & Peanuts

Steam one bag of Broccoli in Microwave. Cut 2 onions into rings. Heat 1 tsp olive oil in medium skillet, fry onion rings, briefly, until light golden. Add one can of tomatoes, stir in 1 tsp cumin, 1 tsp turmeric, ½ tsp cinnamon, a pinch of cayenne pepper. Let simmer for a few minutes. Stir in 1 tablespoon peanut butter and

1 cup Greek yogurt. Add salt to taste and more cayenne pepper, if you like it hot. Fold in broccoli and reheat, if necessary. Sprinkle some chopped lightly salted peanuts on top. Serve with brown rice.

Quick chicken breast

(1) Prepare ahead: slice deboned chicken breast (½ inch), put in microwave safe dish in a single layer and sprinkle with soya sauce (preferably 'light'), marinate for 2 hours or overnight in fridge. Turn slices once, if possible.

(2) Microwave on high for 2 minutes. Turn slices and add 2 more minutes. Proceed like this until fully cooked (juice comes out clear when pierced with a knife) – will take about 5 to 7 minutes all in all.

(3) Add brown rice ('instant' brown rice is ready in 10 minutes) and veggies of your choice (steamed in micro). Don't forget to add turmeric to your rice and other herbs to your veggies (e.g. thyme to beans, sage to peas, oregano to tomatoes, and parsley and garlic to everything).

Quick side dish: Try whole wheat couscous. It's precooked whole wheat, ready in 5 minutes.

Healthy meat loaf

Basis of this dish is ground turkey combined with lots of healthy ingredients:

(1) Combine 1 pound of ground turkey with 2 cups of veggies (carrots, zucchini, bell pepper – whatever you like), 1 large onion, garlic (as much as you like), all kinds of seeds you like (coriander seeds, cumin or caraway seeds, celery seeds) – everything chopped up in your blender – ½ cup of oats (soaked in water, barely covered, for one hour or overnight), and 2 eggs. Add 1 tsp. salt and pepper or chili pepper, if desired. Blend well.

(2) To taste for salt, take one teaspoon of the mixture. Cook in microwave for a few seconds. Sample and add salt, if desired.

(3) Spray a microwave safe dish with cooking spray. Add meatloaf mix and cook for about 15 minutes or until done (depending on microwave).

Serve with another bag of veggies or a salad, rice or mashed potatoes.

If you do not have a lot of time for cooking during your 'normal' day, prepare ahead. This dish may be frozen in order to use for a later meal.

Sauerkraut Salad

Combine barrel cured fermented raw sauerkraut (cut up) with 1 apple, cut into bite size pieces (not peeled), finely chopped onion (you decide how much), add some apple juice, ground or whole cumin/caraway, celery seeds, maybe some ground stevia leaves. Let stand for some minutes. Enjoy!

Sauerkraut *with ground turkey and paprika*

Heat a little bit of vegetable oil in a frying pan; add 1 pound ground turkey, 2 - 3 chopped onions, and some garlic. Stir until turkey is fully cooked. Reduce heat. Stir in 1 tablespoon paprika powder until well blended, add ½ cup of water. Stir in 1 lb of fermented sauerkraut. Let simmer for 5 minutes. Serve with cooked potatoes.

Beets

Beets are easy to cook, but prepare ahead. Cook as whole; otherwise they would "bleed out". After cooling it's easy to peel. Cut into bite size pieces, put in a glass bowl and marinate for a few hours or overnight in a mixture of mustard, vinegar, a pinch of stevia (if you like it slightly sweetened) and salt to taste. Serve cold as a side salad or warm (not hot) as veggies with any meat or fish you like.

Greek Beet Greens and Beet Root Salad

Try to buy really fresh beets with greens at a farmers market. Cook beet roots as mentioned above and cut into bite size pieces. Chop beet greens coarsely. Heat oil in a skillet; add greens. Cook very briefly while stirring until leaves are wilted. In a glass bowl combine greens and root pieces. Toss in juice of 1 lemon and 1 medium onion finely chopped. Peel and squeeze 3 cloves of garlic. Add garlic to 1 cup Greek yogurt, salt to taste. Combine beets and yogurt. Top with walnuts or any other kind of nuts or seeds you like. Serve immediately.

Parsley pesto

Chop parsley leaves (1 cup or more, firmly packed) coarse, transfer to a blender, and add some nuts (walnuts, sunflower seeds, pine nuts) as well as some garlic and blend. Add some olive oil while blending until smooth. This pesto will freshen up steamed fish as well as grilled chicken breast.

Parsley salad

Combine cooked 2 cups quinoa with 4 cups parsley. Add 1 cup cherry tomatoes (halved), finely sliced celery stems, and 2 cloves chopped garlic. Make vinaigrette out of lemon juice (4-5 tablespoons) and olive oil (8 tablespoons), salt and pepper to taste. Sprinkle some walnuts or sunflower seeds on top.

Cooking With Turmeric - Recipe Ideas

Use turmeric as often as possible. Turmeric hardly tastes of anything (only if you use too much, it may taste bitter). Therefore you may use it in any food you do not mind that it turns yellow.

Here are some suggestions:

✓ Yellow rice: add 1 tsp turmeric to water to cook 1 cup of brown rice. Combine with peas for a great side dish.

✓ Color dull looking cauliflower: Either add turmeric to cooking water or – better – cut cauliflower up into small florets, cook in salted water until still firm to bite. Combine in a pan 4 tablespoons butter with ½ teaspoon turmeric, add cayenne pepper, if you like it hot. Place cauliflower in a large dish, drizzle over melted turmeric butter. Add some tomatoes and greens for additional color.

✓ Color your scrambled eggs with some turmeric.

✓ Color your next cake with turmeric – yes: add turmeric to any dough.

✓ Use turmeric in soups and stews.

✓ Add turmeric to your vinaigrette and spice up your salad.

Green Leaves

Turn sautéed greens into something more savory and tender. Use any greens like kale or collard greens – one large bunch. Cut out stems and chop leaves coarsely. Peel and chop 1 medium onion and 3-5 cloves garlic. Heat 1 tablespoon olive oil in medium skillet.

Add onions and garlic to oil and fry for just 1 minute. Add greens and 1 cup of water, broth or white wine to pan. Cover and let simmer for about 5 minutes. Remove cover and cook on high heat until liquid is reduced (about 1 minute). Add about 2 tablespoons red wine or balsamic vinegar. Season to taste with salt, black pepper, and a pinch of cayenne pepper, if you like.

Get Started

Now that you got the idea: Get started. Pick a time for your detox diet. During a period of three weeks you should be able to prepare your meals at home as often as possible and do not have to rely on eating out most of the time. Don't wait for the perfect timing! Figure out how to include all the healthy things and get started right away.

Start on a Monday – this way you will have a weekend to prepare. Banish all tempting foods you should not eat during this period: sweets, soft drinks, sodas, hard liquors.

Even after a few days you will feel energized and healthy! You will like the feeling and it will be easy to stick to the diet – even longer than three weeks.

If you have any questions, visit us on www.yourherbery.com and contact us. We will be happy to assist with any information you need.

Good luck and enjoy your new healthy self!

Note from the Author

My grandmother knew a lot about herbs. She had her knowledge from her mother. She would tell me stories about this woman, who would walk the woods and meadows searching for herbs.

When I was a little girl, she let me play with herbs, cooking for my dolls. And always she would tell me what to look at to identify the specific herb, what these herbs are good for, and how to use them.

Some of the herbal blends I use, are still the recipes of my grandmother. "Sweeter Dreams" is one of these. "Yerba Mate" was her favorite drink in the morning - combined with other herbs you still find in my "Herbal Energy Drink". Dandelion, celery seeds and Green Tea with lemon has been her favorite for detoxifying ("Detox Tea"). But: These days I do not only rely on the knowledge of my grandmother. All information given is scientifically validated.

At one point in my life, I decided to get engaged with herbs again, to help spread the knowledge on herbal benefits for health and wellbeing. I went back to college, got my degree, and started my business. In order to give back, I focus on educating and informing - hopefully making a difference in someone's life.

Dr. Angela C. Fritz

About the Author

Dr. Angela C. Fritz is Vice President of New Medical Frontiers, Inc., Master Herbalist & Holistic Health Practitioner. In 2010 she founded *The Herbery* in order to not only sell herbs, but to provide latest knowledge on the efficacy of herbs for well being. She holds a PHD from the University of Munich, Germany, and is an Academic Member of the American Botanical Council. Dr. Angela C. Fritz started her business career at the University of Vienna, Austria. For 10 years she has been on the management board (CEO) of a major newspaper company in Vienna Austria.

>>><<<

New Medical Frontiers, Inc. was founded in January 1999 by Dr. Mark Fritz, NMD. The focus is on documentation, information and education in the field of Natural Medicine. Today this company has a huge database documenting latest and up-to-date scientific research carried out at renowned U.S. and international medical schools and research institutions. Visit us at newmedicalfrontiers.com.

The Herbery is a branch of New Medical Frontiers, Inc. It is the place, where you can buy heirloom remedy blends, dried herbs, herbal teas, and essential oils, and learn more about herbs and their health benefits. Visit us at www.yourherbery.com.

www.ingramcontent.com/pod-product-compliance
Lightning Source LLC
Chambersburg PA
CBHW050557280326
41933CB00011B/1875